FREEDUM

FREEDOM

Feeling Your Way Through Chronic Fatigue Syndrome

FAITH CANTER

EMPOWERED
BOOKS

Published in 2020 by Empowered Books

ISBN Paperback: 978-0-9957047-6-3
Ebook: 978-0-9957047-7-0

Published with the help of Indie Authors World

www.indieauthorsworld.com

IndieAuthors
World

DEDICATION

Dear Toon,

Thank you for showing many deeper ways to freedom

Thank you for the lessons, the laughter and the heartaches

Thank you for the connection, the release and the love

Thank you for teaching me truths and freeing me.

With Love,

Faith xx

CONTENTS

INTRODUCTION

My story of Chronic Fatigue Syndrome (CFS) is a fairly standard one it seems.

It began when I was fairly young with depression, anxiety and a few obsessive compulsive behaviours (which later developed into OCDs). Perhaps this was brought on by some unhappy experiences I had as a child, such as child abuse, or learned from family, or from feeling the early pressures of society wanting me to do better, do more and conform. I feel it was a combination of all the above. Everything I did had a tinge of people-pleasing, perfectionism, over-achieving to it. I did not feel enough in the world and felt I had to work hard to be what I thought would make me enough, liked, loved and noticed. I pushed and pulled and pretended and I was used and abused, and I hated who I was on almost every level. I had eating disorders, I started cutting myself, I binged on food, drink, drugs, people, cleaning, anything to distract myself from the thoughts in my own head.

For many years it was like this; I was suffering with chronic back and head pain, severe IBS and food intolerances, and constantly ill with whatever was doing the rounds. Oh, and I was really mentally and physically exhausted.

Eventually, many years later, I got salmonella poisoning in India and was ill for a very long time. When I returned to the UK, I then got glandular fever and that was the straw that finally broke the camel's back and I unknowingly (at the time) found myself with CFS.

It took almost two years of many doctor's visits, tests and private consultants to rule out every other thing it could possibly be before I finally accepted the diagnoses of CFS. I knew from others I had met along the way while researching all the possible illnesses I could have, that CFS was not one you'd find much help for. Many are told to go home and wait for it to pass or just given anti-depressants and painkillers to help with the symptoms and some are told they'll never recover. I could not accept this, so I did everything within my power to find out if I could possibly have something else that I could recover from. As soon as I accepted this diagnosis however I got worse because I gave up, I got more depressed and I did not know what to do or who to turn to.

One day I was in pieces, bordering on hysterical (again), while reading more CFS horror stories that a well-meaning, but really unhelpful CFS charity liked to send out regularly to its subscribers. At that point, my then husband found me and basically ordered me to stop doing this to myself. And you know what? He was right, I was doing this to myself. I couldn't do much back then, but I didn't have to make myself feel worse by reading this stuff. So, I made it my mission to read every recovery story I could, from any illness, accident or trauma I could find. I found that people had made full recoveries from terminal cancer, HIV, being paralysed and told they'd never walk again, and even come back from the dead and similar things like this. I thought, if they could recover from these things then I could recover from CFS.

I read story after story of people recovering from CFS. They all used slightly different approaches but all with some core elements as their foundation. These elements are the ones I share within this book - of course. These elements are also the ones that, if addressed when you are just in the chronic fatigue stage of your journey, before it even gets to CFS itself, can prevent it from escalating to the syndrome stage.

Many people will tell you that you cannot recover from CFS or that the people that apparently have, then obviously didn't have it in the first place. I can tell you I had every single NHS and private test and consultation I could find in the UK and they all said the same thing - CFS! Let those people have their beliefs, yours don't have to be the same. You can recover from many things people say you cannot recover from; just start searching for all the thousands of stories of recovery out there and see for yourself.

Life is meant to be for living, for thriving, not for just surviving ad sedating. If you don't feel this way and are becoming more disillusioned, exhausted and overwhelmed, then these are life's whispers to make a change. Not next year, five years from now or when you retire - now! Because when we do not listen to the whispers, eventually they become screams. And this is when something like CFS comes along, it's the body screaming for change.

I believe Chronic Fatigue Syndrome, (like many illnesses), is a symptom of society being ill, not us. We are just doing our best to fit into a society that does not work and makes us feel like we need fixing when it's not ourselves at all that need fixing. CFS can and will be one of your greatest teachers; the question is, will you allow it, or will you fight it?

CHAPTER 1

LISTEN TO YOURSELF

I would like to make a note right here, very clearly at the beginning of this book...

I AM NOT a doctor, consultant or trained specialist in Chronic Fatigue Syndrome. I have never said I am, and my words and knowledge are not being shared with you from that viewpoint.

What I am, however, is someone that lived and breathed CFS for far too long because not one of the practitioners I went to see in the years I was chronically ill and bedbound, had more than a vague clue about CFS themselves. They really had no idea where it came from, why it hung around or why or how someone got better or not.

In the time I lived with this illness and due to being financially in a good place at that time, I tried every single private consultant I could find and every single pill, potion, lotion and alternative treatment out there to become well again. There are very few things I did not try, either from standard medical professionals or later more natural routes.

In the years since becoming well, I trained in all the modalities that I believed assisted me on my journey to full health, and taught others who were struggling with this condition, to help them along their path to full health too.

One of the few positive outcomes of living with CFS is that it teaches us to listen to ourselves, our own bodies. When we really start to do that, our mental and physical health returns to us.

So, although I share a lot of things within the pages of this book, I urge you, above all else, to listen to yourself. What feels right to you? How does your body feel when you do a certain thing? Are you drained after doing a certain other thing? Does it put you in more conflict? Does it cause you mental or physical pain?

Everyone's journey is different, we all came to be here from different pasts, but the common thread among it all is that when we really start to feel and listen to our own bodies, our own self-knowledge things really start to change (and this can apply, not just when suffering from CFS, but with many other illnesses and hardships we find in our path).

No one diet is right for everyone, no pill, potion, lotion, supplement or treatment "fixes" it all. But your body knows what's best for you and when you learn to listen to it, the conflict which keeps you feeling caged inside a body that is against you, starts to fade away.

Listen to the whispers, your body knows what's best for you!

CHAPTER 2

IT'S NOT YOU THAT'S UNWELL, IT'S THE WORLD!

After I was free of CFS, someone I knew who was still unwell with CFS, once said to me that if I still had to continue doing the things that got me well from CFS, then I was not healed from it. I said I could not possibly agree less.

Why? Because it is not really us that is unwell but the world. We become unwell because we are trying to fit into a sick world. This world is crazy unwell! We are born into a society that turns away from the heart and instead, rests firmly in the head. What I mean is that when we are small children, we do not care what we look like, what we are wearing or what we sing or dance like, we are totally heart-centred and happy. But, as we grow, society tells us we need to be quiet, conform and fit in.

As such, we start learning we need to be something other than ourselves, something more, something acceptable. We become head-centred and unhappy with who we are. As we grow with age, the need to "be more" grows alongside. We are set tests, exams, given merits, certificates, rewards and guidance to be a greater version of us, the one who will be finally happy, who will have the money, the partner, the house and fulfilment. Always a carrot dangling, always the next thing or things, but never quite there... well, not for very long, but that next thing of things is waiting for us and that one will help us along... apparently.

We feel greater pressure and overwhelm, that we are not "enough" and we meet more and deeper sources of unhappiness. We are always searching for a way to fix, change or improve our mood, situation, life or even soul. Lost and drowning, yet trying to save face, to fit in and be whatever it is we've been told we need to to be happy.

As this continues, our mental health deteriorates. There may be times when we feel great. A new distraction has come along and new way to feel great, to fit in and find happiness. But mostly it does not last and again we are left feeling like we are the only one in the world this s@#t does not work for. Great! Just great!

The years of pretending may pass by, but we know the truth. This is not real life, we are surviving (just about) not thriving, like everyone else appears to do.

Then something comes along to shake things up, an illness or an issue we need to deal with somewhere, and we realise there is indeed another way, and that just because it appeared to be the norm to behave in this way, it is not the way we wish to live any more. Things can be different. But of course we have been thinking a certain way for most of our lives and it's sometimes hard in that "big-bad-world" to remember what we have learned, that we don't have to jump through hoops to be happy, we just have to follow our hearts.

So, you see, to remain sane in some sort of way in this crazy-ass-world, we need to keep doing at least some of the things we learned in our journey to freedom in the first place. We need to ensure we harness the healing powers of life and don't slip back into feeling dead from trying to live in a society that seems to love to create pressure, "not enoughness" and toxicity at every turn.

So, we can choose. We can choose to either live in a cave on a remote mountainside away from others, meditating eighteen hours a day, or we can choose to develop healing skills and habits that we harness to be able to live happy, healthy lives in this crazy place we currently call "life".

You are not unwell. You have learned you needed to be something you are not, in order to fit into a society full of people who are all trying to be something they are not, too. The world is unwell, not you. In fact, you were so good at trying to fit into this crazy-ass-world, you won the gold star for it, you excelled at it, you made yourself unwell to fit in with it!

But now it's time to use your ill health to learn the lessons needed to thrive in this poorly world, rather than being sucked under by it.

CHAPTER 3

THE IMPORTANCE OF WORKING WITH THE MIND

When I first started my journey to full health, I focused almost solely on healing my body - I mean, it was my body that felt so incredibly awful after all. I had put my body through so much over the years that I knew it needed a lot of support and cleansing. I detoxed my diet, my body, my cosmetics, cleaning products, home, garden, animals, even my then husband. I did it all. I felt worse at these times because I was releasing a lot of toxins from a lifetime of bad foods, booze, drugs and chemicals in and around me. But, after the initial detox symptoms faded, I always felt a little better.

There is no doubt in my mind that all our bodies are toxic from the way we live our lives these days, however just reducing and removing these physical toxins alone will not lead to full health. In fact, those who focus on this alone are the ones who seem to relapse most of the time.

It is essential for any plan, programme, diet, detox or life change you make (even if you do not have CFS) to be one of combined physical and mental change.

If you do the mental "work" alongside the physical work, then it makes the physical stuff easier and longer lasting. But the main thing is that it means we generally don't go back to where we began time and time again.

For instance, research suggests that 97% of people who go on diets put the weight back on, and sometimes more. This is generally because we don't do the mental work when we stop eating junk food. We don't address why we are eating like that, what needs it is fulfilling in us, whether it comes from a lack of self-love, or any trauma or abuse this is covering up. So we just go right back to doing those same things again after we have lost all the weight.

It's a little bit the same with CFS. We have many reasons why we first got ill; yes, toxicity of the body is part of it and certainly adds to our burden. But for most, it started originally with the mind. If, like me and every other person with CFS I have met, you were a chronic overthinking person, or burning the candle at both ends, a people-pleaser, an achiever, a trauma sufferer, victim, depressive, anxious, stress-head - then over the years this has built up and caused a highly sensitive nervous system that is constantly on high alert and in the "fight-or-flight" response mode.

Being here for prolonged periods of time leads to the nervous system drawing resources from and eventually shutting down other systems of the body. So, you start to have many physical issues too. You are fatigued, in pain, have IBS, hormonal issues, lymphatic concerns, you ache, itch and become sensitive to light, sound, smells, chemicals, food and many other previously harmless things.

So, to become fully well and healthy again, the mind needs help. Not just starting a few meditation classes (although this is a great start), but real assistance to break habits of thinking, realising half the stresses are imagined, realising we have a choice over what we are thinking, becoming OK with being human, making friends with our thoughts and learning not to be triggered so much by this crazy-ass-world.

Yes, there may also be some deeper stuff to resolve from past trauma or family issues, however just learning to love being in your own head and life again are the key.

This reduces our conflict which then reduces our nervous system responses to every little thing, which in turn reduces our physical symptoms and puts the body into a healing place. The less conflicted we are, the more easily the body removes toxins, the better the endocrine system works, the more energy we have, the clearer our thinking becomes and the less pain we feel. We can even start to eat and do things we had considered highly toxic in our recovery, and not be as affected by these things, because mentally we are in a good place, so these things flow much easier through us.

When we are in a bad place mentally, we are like a magnet to all the toxic things around us. When we are in a good place mentally, it's like we have a forcefield surrounding us and things just bounce right off, or pass through us with a little more ease.

It's all about the mind, because when the mind is strong the body becomes strong too.

CHAPTER 4

WHY DO PEOPLE HAVE PHYSICAL SYMPTOMS THEN?

As you may have guessed, I am no scientist, nor do I have any interest in being one. However, as I understand it, when we keep triggering our nervous system, we keep activating our fight-or-flight response, as we become fearful of our own thoughts, of what we imagine others think of us, about our health concerns, our bodies, our lives and our "not being enoughs". When we do this long-term, it's hard for our body to deal with, it needs to draw on resources from other parts of the body to remain vigilant over what it has decided is a threat to us. As it does this, other parts of the body start to act up, digestive and hormonal issues likely come along, and usually some immune and lymphatic problems too.

I always used to wonder why everyone I met with CFS had digestive issues and this is the reason why. The body needs to draw resources away from the digestive system to maintain its high-alert position within the nervous system. Doctors often comment on IBS being stress-related and it is because the nervous system is triggered too frequently, which has a direct impact on the digestive system. This is also why most things we do to help our digestive system at a physical level only help it for short periods of time and not for the long-term, because we are not addressing the under-lying nervous system over-stimulation issue. Obviously, changing things physically whilst still in the stimulated place can help, but they do not 'fix' what is going on.

For years I did not allow myself to eat many, many foods. I ate lots of ferments, did a yeast and parasite cleanse and many other things and believed I had "fixed" my digestive issues. But that was not the case because I still could not eat some basic healthy foods (I am not counting wheat and sugars and rubbish like that, which we should not really be eating anyway). No, the real healing came when I addressed my nervous system triggers, the way I felt about myself, my body and my life – in short, my thoughts.

All the other stuff I did was amazingly helpful, (and still is to maintain a healthy, balanced body in a crazy toxic world), and meant my IBS was about 80% reduced. But the physical body stuff alone will never heal anything completely by itself long-term, you must address the mind stuff too, no matter what you are struggling with.

So, why do you have physical symptoms then? Because you have been triggering the nervous system to extremes for too long and it's run out of resources and searching for them elsewhere. Plus it's in super-high-alert all the time and sees most things as a threat.

Also, when the digestive system is impaired, (as it will be in this heightened triggered place), it will reduce your uptake of nutrients substantially, because the digestive system isn't working at 100% capacity as that energy is needed elsewhere, which therefore has an impact on other areas of the body. This is the same for other systems in the body that start to become compromised by being constantly on high alert. Therefore, seemingly unrelated symptoms start to pop up and become an issue. They are not unrelated at all and it seems in most cases, it is not possible to be fixed by the pills, potions and lotions prescribed for these concerns because in fact, they are all being caused (or at the very least exaggerated) by the mind and its long-term heightened nervous system response.

CHAPTER 5

FOCUS ON WHAT YOU CAN DO INSTEAD OF WHAT YOU CANNOT

It's so very easy with CFS, (and I would imagine many other chronic illnesses), to focus on what we cannot do. I remember it vividly. I would spend a good proportion of my day focused on not being able to work, walk the dogs, look after my husband, clean the house, cook food, go out partying etc. But guess what? This does not help us and in fact makes us much, much worse. Why? Because every time we put our attention on what we cannot do, we reinforce those very things in our lives, and more importantly, in our bodies, because we trigger a nervous system response.

Chemical changes start to happen to reinforce the very things we focus on within our bodies. So, rather than focusing on what we do not want and reinforcing these things, let's do our best to focus on what we do want and reinforce those things instead. Instead of thinking of all the great many things we cannot do any more, let's focus on the small number of things we can.

We may be able to have a bath today... result! Not only will we clean our physical body, but we will have super-relaxing and nurturing - bonus! We can also make it more healing if we wish, with things like adding a mug of Epsom salts to the hot water (high in magnesium, which many people are deficient in - it draws out toxins and muscle aches and pains).

Or, we may manage to do the washing-up this morning, so that's one less thing for our partner/friend/carer to do.

It's OK to take baby steps.   We may start to sort out our accounts, or make an appointment with the bank /dentist/ doctor/hairdresser. Whatever we have managed to do, pat ourselves on the back for it. Today is a good day!

I know full well this isn't always as easy as it sounds, but just do your best with what you have got and above all else, don't give yourself a hard time if you slip up. This is totally pointless and that "giving yourself a hard time" triggers the nervous system worse than the original issue. Just remember you are human and the habit of focusing on what you cannot do has been a long-standing one. This new and healthier habit may just take a little bit of time to override the previous one.

It may be a good idea for you to write down at the end of each day, the things you are happy you did, just three things:

Today I am happy that I...

took a shower and got dressed

put the washing on

did the washing up

put the rubbish out

made that appointment

dusted my cabinet

unloaded the dishwasher

made it downstairs

finished reading that book

spoke to a friend/sent those emails

put a food order in

didn't scream at someone/didn't lose my s#1t

was there for a friend/sent a card

meditated/tapped/yoga/visualized

took my supplements/made a green smoothie

body brushed

sat in the garden/looked out the window for a while...

whatever pleases you to have been able to do with your day.

The more we focus on what we can and have achieved, the more we are able to do those things because we are not triggering the nervous system response. That makes it a whole heap easier to then do more of the nice things because we are not as mentally and physically drained.

CHAPTER 6

HOW CAN I REDUCE MY CONFLICT RIGHT NOW?

This is the ultimate healing question for anyone with a chronic illness, or even low yet persistent levels of stress and fatigue.

I invite you to write that question on Post-it notes, or set it as a reminder in your phone, journal regularly or remember to ask yourself daily in some way or another. This one question stops the pushing, pleasing, fixing, changing, improving, overwhelm and most importantly stressing.

Whatever it is you are in an overly-stimulated mind set about right now can be reduced by this simple question. Maybe ask yourself out loud.

It's likely you are in conflict about your health or maybe it's your finances, or perhaps your appointments, friends, family or chores. Whatever you are feeling conflicted about, without a shadow of a doubt, will not under any circumstance get any better from continuing to get all conflicted about it. It does not help one ounce! Not one!

However, what could help is you consciously putting yourself into a less conflicted space, because then you'll have much more mental and physical capacity to deal with whatever is going on. It's not going to make your health worse (thus making the situation worse) and you will see a clear way through whatever is happening when you are more open and in flow. You cannot be open and in flow when you are fighting yourself and life. The two do not co-exist.

So, whenever you feel the struggle of the mind, ask yourself: "How can I reduce my conflict right now?" There is also a slight variation of this that works well when you really must do the thing you are conflicted about: "How can I do this in a less conflicted way?".

Your response to either of these questions could be a physical activity: breathe/ get some fresh air/meditate/ tap/journal, or say to yourself: remember I can choose not to feel this way/it's OK to feel this way/it's OK to be human/take some time out/let it go/it's OK to be human/ it's OK to walk away/make a plan/get it out of my head/ it's OK to feel/what's this inviting me to do or be more of?/ move into my heart etc.

Add this question to your Thriving Guide (more about this later). Put reminders in and on anything you can. This one question will save your sanity and thus your health many times over.

CHAPTER 7
WHEN YOU TRY NOT TO FEEL, YOU DON'T HEAL

This may seem like a strange thing to say when everyone is telling us always that we must be positive, say positive affirmations or mantras, think only positive thoughts etc. I fell into this trap too. I thought if I could block the bad thoughts, then I would stop feeling depressed, anxious and overwhelmed and then I would stop triggering my nervous system that made all my symptoms much worse.

In fact, initially I did move forward in my recovery by using various techniques to just think positively. But I soon realised I was stagnating. I had improved but the improvements only went so far, and although I was trying to be positive, I was far from happy. In fact, I even went as far as to try hypnotherapy and a few other modalities to "find my happy". I thought maybe if I could be happy, then I could fully recover. I just did not know how to access this happy place.

It was then I came across the work of Sandy Newbigging (Hay House author of "Mind Calm" and various other amazing books) and realised what I had been doing. In my bid to stay positive and be happy I was pushing away parts of myself. I was deeply scared of these parts because in the past, they had taken me time and time again to such dark and scary places that I did not want to let them in again. I could not keep going there as some day I might not find my way back again.

We cannot push away the "bad" and expect to only feel the "good", it doesn't work like that. We must learn to accept all the parts of us there are. This way the "bad" stuff does not have power over us and the "good" stuff has space to flow.

Sandy's work taught me that it's OK to feel, in fact we should encourage it. It's OK to feel "bad" and when we are OK with it being there, it loses its power. But what we do is label it "bad" and want it to go away, or we start to believe our stories of why it is bad and in turn, we are bad. But, when we realise these are just stories, and that we do in fact have a choice to believe them or not - they fade away.

Our minds can be crazy scary places, or we can see them as they really are: amazing, brilliant indicators that something is off and we are being invited to make a change.

So, instead of all of a sudden feeling things like "Why did he treat me this way? I must be such a s#@t person", we can see that this situation/relationship/thing is not meant for us (otherwise it would be right and good and happening) and that life is inviting a redirection rather than rejecting us. And, there is nothing wrong with us at all, life is showing us what is right for us instead.

We must acknowledge the bad to feel the directions of life's guidance for us. We must feel the bad to know when to let go. And, we have to feel the bad to know how to feel the good. If you never felt bad, how would you know what happy was?

This is a technique I find extremely helpful when I wake up and instantly feel sad/worried/upset/angry/hurt/trig-gered/emotional/pained. Rather than searching for its source and blaming it all on that person/event/memory (which feeds into a prepared story of why my life is s#@t), I allow myself to be with that feeling. I allow myself to be with that part of me, to lean into it, to learn from it.

I close my eyes and imagine myself opening to this feel-ing, embracing these emotions. I invite this feeling into my heart and body, I welcome it in, even hug it, telling it that it's OK to be there and I'm not going to push it away any longer. I fully embrace this feeling in myself, feeling it in every cell, welcoming home part of me that has been shut out. It holds no power over me in this moment as I accept it being there.

In this moment, when I am not fighting it, I am often gifted with insights of why it's really there. Not the prepared story of all the times gone by, but the one that says something like "Whatever you are seeking on the outside is really what you first need to give yourself within" and other such insightful guru type things, ha!

Anything we fight within ourselves keeps us where we don't want to be. When we can learn to be with ourselves like this, we stop reinforcing the very things we don't want in our lives.

Fighting creates conflict within us, which in turn triggers the nervous system response that makes all our symptoms much worse.

To heal from our trauma, stress, life choices and health concerns, we need to reduce our daily conflict, but to do that we need to be OK with it being there, so that we don't fuel it into being more of the very thing we don't want.

That feeling you are feeling now... maybe you're feeling sceptical/confused/unsure/overwhelmed - allow it to be there. Don't ignore it or push it away. Feel it now. Close your eyes and imagine yourself embracing it, maybe hugging it or inviting it into your heart. Allow its presence, honour its humanness within you and embody its being in every cell. As you breathe, breathe it in, accept it, tell it it's OK to be here and you'll not push it away any more. Do this for however long feels right, but until you feel it all. Take a few deep breaths, fully embracing it, and then open your eyes and come back to where you are now.

How does that feel?

For me, it's always like coming home. There is an ease and peace there.

Here's a little reminder though, we are not accepting our "story" about the feeling, that's something made up in our mind from all our previous experiences. What we are doing is accepting the feeling itself, the raw emotion without anything else mind-based attached to it.

What are you feeling now?

Feel that feeling like we have described above, experiment with it, welcome it home and feel yourself creating a space of health and healing within rather than one of dis-ease.

CHAPTER 8

YOU HAVE THOUGHT TOO MUCH, NOT DONE TOO MUCH!

Most of the time, (but not all), it's not that you have done too much that creates a crash or blip, it's that you have thought too much about it.

Let me illustrate:

A letter about a hospital appointment comes through for a date in a month's time. Whilst reading the information about the appointment, you start to think about all the things you need to do for it, eg:

➢ make sure nothing else is booked in the diary within a few days either side of the appointment

➢ tell your carer

➢ arrange a driver or arrange for someone to go with you

➢ tell the hospital you need assistance

➢ make sure you have food and drink with you

➢ ask your doctor if you should take anything/do anything extra

> ➢ write a list of the things to remember to ask on the
> day there in case you forget, etc.

Instantly you have gone into over-thinking, which leads to low-level anxiety and stress which triggers your nervous system.

As the appointment gets nearer, you haven't heard back from all of the above people so you worry and get anxious about this all the more.

It's a week before the appointment now and you are anxious about how going out of the house and being in a stressful, busy and noisy environment is going to affect you.

It's two days before the appointment, you think you have remembered everything, but have you? You check your lists again and check arrangements with others. You must make sure it's all exactly right to make the most of the appointment and to reduce the stress and exhaustion going out of the house will cause.

The day of the appointment, you did not sleep well because you were worried about it. What if what they say is bad news, or you must take new medicines or do something else, or what if they decide you are better than you are and take away your benefits?

Before even leaving the house, you are now very anxious and exhausted.

The hospital environment is very stimulating, as you suspected, and you are feeling worse. You have to have conversations with people, be polite and then the doctor has lots to say and ask, you are trying to keep it all together, answer properly and remember the questions you wanted to ask.

After what seems like hours, you can leave, you wait for the driver to take you home. They are cheery and chatting and all you want to do it fall in a heap and rest, but you must keep going for a bit longer, but you feel awful and this is all too much.

You finally get home and fall onto the bed, exhausted. But you cannot rest, your mind is wired, you are thinking about everything the doctor said and what he did not say and what you forgot to ask even though you had a list.

You are angry with the doctor and/or yourself for something that was or wasn't said.

You worry about how this trip is going to affect you over the coming days. You have an appointment in three or four days' time with someone about something, will you be OK by then? What if you are not? Do you have a back-up plan? Can you ask so-and-so to do something for you in case?

You fall asleep eventually, totally exhausted and hoping you feel better when you wake.

When you wake you feel the same and you worry you have really overdone it this time. You think that maybe you just shouldn't go to hospital appointments or you should cancel your appointment in a few days' time.

Why do you feel like this? It's not fair. This should not exhaust you that much, you haven't really done that much, etc.

And thus, the crash is here! The more you worry about crashing, the more it happens, because you keep triggering the nervous system response and you feel more and more exhausted, achy, pained and foggy.

You see, hardly any of this was the actual "doing", it was the over-thinking of the doing. Yes, you may have moved around more than you are used to, however it was all that worry leading up to, whilst there, and afterwards which was the real trigger for the crash.

People often ask me to help them to find and maintain a baseline for physical activity. My response is always: your baseline is whatever you can do without going into the heightened overactivity of thoughts about your physical activity. I have even seen people go into this thinking about finding their baseline.

Our aim is to do our daily things (and the odd extras like hospital appointments etc.) in a non-conflicted way. When we can do this, we stop triggering the nervous system in a way that it affects our physical bodies and output.

If the above hospital example resonates with you, then I invite you to start tapping (explained at the back of the book) or journalling as soon as you receive the first trigger (in this case, the letter from the hospital) to get these thoughts out and addressed. I then invite you to ask yourself, "How can I do this thing in a non-conflicted way?"

Maybe make a plan or write lists so you can organise everything way ahead of time. Ask yourself: "Do I need to do this at all? Can someone assist me?" and lastly, but most importantly, remind yourself that this stressful over-thinking is made up in your head and as such, you can choose not to think it. "I can choose not to reinforce the overwhelm/stress/anxiety, I can choose another way." Take some deep breaths and remember that it is not the "doing" but the "thinking" that may cause a blip or even a crash.

This same way of thinking translates into daily activities indoors, as well as things like hospital appointments or social gatherings. If you think to yourself you'd like to do some painting today, or wash the dishes, or take a shower, but then you spend two hours thinking about how much energy that would take, how tired you could be afterwards and all the whats, buts and maybes that could happen, then almost certainly you will feel both mentally and physically exhausted because you have overthought the whole thing. Then you'll possibly say things to yourself like, "See, I can't even paint/wash/shower any more without being totally wiped out", when this is not actually the case. It was all that over-thinking/worry/stress about the "doing" before, during and after that causes the mental and physical exhaustion from it.

Try this one for size: you are thinking about painting/ washing/showering now and you just get up and do it as soon as you have the thought. No other thoughts about it, just do it. It's over and done with within twenty minutes and you can sit back down and rest right afterwards.

Do you best, where possible, to get into this habit of just doing rather than worrying about things. We create these mountains in our minds and then wonder why we are so exhausted from them.

I used to do this myself: the idea of going upstairs was always my mountain. It was such hard work that whenever I made it downstairs, I'd worry for the rest of the day about going upstairs again (rather than celebrating making it downstairs!) By the time I did go up the stairs, I could barely make it and would lay exhausted either on the bed or the bathroom floor until I felt able to move again. Yes, my muscles and body were not strong, but they were weakened substantially more by my thoughts about the mountain I had to climb.

Do your best not to create mountains out of your daily moments and then they will pass by more easily as these moments really should.

CHAPTER 9
START AFRESH NOW

What came before this point no longer matters, it's moot, void, obsolete. It's fact, or at least your interpretation of fact, and that is all.

What I mean by this is that often when we have lost our way, our sense of being, our equilibrium and balance, we give ourselves a hard time for being lost. I noticed this particularly when I started along the alternative path I now find myself on. Because I now knew myself better, I knew the teachings, techniques and theory, I worried that if I lost my way, I would mentally beat myself up about this. How had this happened again? Why? When's it going to stop... etc?

The thing is we just go around in mental circles when we do this. We make the original things we were sucked under by almost irrelevant because we start giving ourselves a hard time for being in a hard place and then simply being human and losing our way.

It's OK to be in that hard place. It may not be nice or where you'd like to be hanging out, but once you are out of that hard place, don't let yourself get dragged back down.

What came before this moment, even if it was just an hour or a day, even a week or month of dwelling in that dark place, it has been, it's gone and it's done with, fact. Let it go, move on, start afresh right now!

It serves neither you nor anyone else to keep dwelling on where you were and that you should have known better. You didn't know better that time, but you might do next time, if you don't wear yourself out both mentally and physically going over what a bad healer you are.

Plan how to help yourself next time you are hanging out on the verge of that dark place, maybe use the Thriving Guide (mentioned in Chapter 35 of this book) - but let it go.

What came before is fact, but it does not have to be your future too.

It's done, now it's time to move on!

CHAPTER 10

WHAT ARE YOU REINFORCING WITH YOUR THOUGHTS?

A better way of asking this question is: "What are my thoughts fuelling?"

Not only does constantly worrying about, over-thinking and over-analysing things trigger the nervous system and thus make you feel both mentally and physically worse, it also does something else. Because our minds do not know the difference between something real or something made up, when we focus a lot on negative things, or things that have not even happened, our mind responds as if it believes it's actually happening. The mind generates chemical changes throughout the body to address this persistent trigger. Then the body has to address having too much adrenaline running through it. It's not natural to be in this fight-or-flight response long term so the body is trying to eliminate the adrenaline as it would if you were actually in a fight or flee situation and running away from something scary. This causes physical symptoms and thus makes your CFS worse.

So, when we keep focusing on those things, we reinforce the very things we do not want in our lives.

A better way of addressing what's happening within us would be to allow your body to feel the symptom and not fight it. Just allow it to be present and part of you. When you don't fuel it with your thoughts, it does not grow so much because you are not in that nervous response as much. When you allow it to just be, it has no power over you and your health. And often, it will reduce by itself.

Just allowing things to be may not heal you, but it sure as hell won't add to your already overburdened nervous system and health.

When we focus on our fears, we fuel our fears, but when we focus on our fun, we can fuel that too! Choose wisely where your focus goes and if it goes to fears, then at least don't give yourself a hard time for being human and just let that blip go and move on.

CHAPTER 11

IT'S NOT THE PROBLEM THAT'S THE PROBLEM, BUT THE WAY YOU THINK ABOUT IT THAT IS

We've all got problems, right? And it feels like those problems are the cause of all our stress, anxiety, unhappiness and ill health. Well, really, they are not.

It's your way of thinking about these problems that really is the issue.

You see, you may have an issue with your ex-partner or your health or work or something else, and that may be an instant trigger for you when it happens and makes you feel stressed. This is a totally normal human reaction. However, we then allow the problem to play out again and again. We doubt what we said or they said, we should have said this, why did they say that, this isn't true, that isn't right, and all this self questioning. We blame ourselves and we blame others, we feel victims to how others choose to treat us, we get upset, distressed, angry and sad. It's at this point that the problem is no longer the problem - we are!

It's our thinking about the problem that is now making us stressed, upset, angry and ill, not the original problem. It's all self-made now, (unless someone is standing in front of you, still shouting at you or demanding something of you), then the stress is now all your own doing.

Once a trigger, (whether it's a particular ongoing issue or an argument or misunderstanding), has passed, we can then choose if we are going to allow the event to continue to affect our mental and physical health. We really do have the choice.

Everything used to stress me out, I felt like everything was a personal attack on me, even when things happened at work. My life felt like one big stress: everyone wanted a piece of me, I had to sort out everyone else's mess and to top it off, I had all this personal stuff going on too. Yes, people did and said unhelpful things and yes, I was an HR Manager which can be a very taxing role. However, it was me that would not let things go, who felt the victim, that went over and over things and took all my stresses home with me. That was all me!

It's not about just trying to forget about stuff with that large glass of wine, a TV boxset or a shopping spree; it's about remembering that the way you think about things builds them up out of proportion.

So, if you remind yourself that, yes, that person may have been an arsehole, but you are not going to allow their arsehole-ness to affect your life and health, you are going to let it go, then you will find you can, in fact, let things go. That person no longer has control over you then, as they did before. No matter if you have been used or abused, if you keep re-running the problem, then it's you that is allowing them further control of your life. They aren't doing anything any more - you are! You, I am sorry to say, are doing it to yourself.

The problem is only a problem when it first triggers you. After that point, you have a choice to let go of the problem and the person who caused it, and thus their hold of your life goes too. Or else, you can choose to hold on, replay it, dwell on it and blame it for all your mental and physical health issues and bad luck thereafter, when in fact, that is most likely all your own doing.

Remember, every time you allow your dwelling on a problem to run away with itself, you trigger that nervous system response, so let's not allow other people or events to have any such hold over our health moving forward.

CHAPTER 12

GET IT OUT OF YOUR HEAD

G et all that nonsense, those crazy thoughts, that over-thinking, planning, analysing, replaying - whatever it is, get it out.

Every single person I have met with CFS is an over-thinker. We think about the past, the present, the future, things that will never happen, things that should have happened but didn't, and things that are not important at all. We go around and around in circles with it, adding to our stress load as we go.

When we are over-thinking things, getting stressed and anxious, we really notice the difference in our physical health; we feel more tired, less able to sleep and all our other physical symptoms like sensitivities and pain are worse. We can see a direct correlation between stress and health. We see this because it's easy to feel it when we trigger the nervous system in such a strong way.

The thing is, because you are in a heightened level of stress, because of your illness, you don't always notice what is keeping you at that baseline of stress, because you are not feeling worse, but for some reason you are also not getting much better.

This baseline of stress or the nervous system response is fuelled by your over-thinking and is most noticeable in you during the later stages of recovery, or when you feel you are fully recovered and want to start working or going going out into the world again. This is almost always why you relapse once you have been well for a while.

What I mean by this is that when you don't address how your mind deals with day-to-day life (and the normal stresses, plans and events that living in this crazy-ass-triggering-world throw at us), then the thoughts begin to take over again. You begin to feel overwhelmed, stuck, anxious, scared and thus ill again.

I remember clearly when in my later stages of recovery that each time I started wanting to do more again, (social-ise, blog, create my own business, work etc.), I started to feel overwhelmed and that would start to have a very nega-tive impact on my health. The more well I felt physically, the worse I would end up feeling mentally, and before long, the physical stuff would kick in. It was because I was trying to be be more, do more, achieve more again. That old over-everything-er person would re-appear and then suddenly it would all be too much again. In my head I'd be screaming, "Retreat, retreat, it's all getting too much again!" but on the outside I'd be saying things like "I can do this", "I am well", "it's all good", etc. And then a crash would come.

One of the keys to not feeling overwhelmed again during or after recovery is to get it out of your head. Generally, people with CFS are "over-everything-ers"; we are trying to be, do or achieve more. We generally feel pretty good at multi-tasking as we can think about a lot of things at once. But this is what helped to get us ill. However if we are good at multi-tasking, if worked with properly, it can assist us with our recovery and future plans, even our life, because it does come naturally to us. It does not have to be something we have to "get rid of" to become well, just something that needs a little guidance.

So, use this crazy brain to assist your life rather than let it assist you into overwhelm and ill health. Get the ideas out, any way that feels good to you, but get them out. The moment you start to have a lot of plans, feel overwhelmed, confused, over-worked, get them all out. Every single option/idea/plan, all the parts of it, everything.

Here is an example of how I make this work for me.

I have often found it difficult to remain totally present during meditation when I have new projects on the go. Ideas keep coming up and demanding attention in some way. So, unlike most meditators I know, I have a pen and pad next to the place I meditate. If something super-important or a wonderful idea comes to mind, rather than playing this game with myself of attempting not to interact with the thought, but also not wanting to forget it, I open one eye during the meditation and quickly scribble the idea down on my pad and then close my eyes and go back to a much more peaceful meditation.

When it's out, it's no longer causing you conflict. You are no longer trying to remember everything, think of all the parts of the plan or what could go right or wrong, and you can see your ideas and all their parts very clearly.

My three favourite ways to get the thoughts out are as follows (brain-dumping is the best one for plans/work stuff – just so you know):

Brain-Dumping: *I like to dump all my ideas/plans etc. onto paper. I draw spider diagrams of my idea or group of similar ideas. I write the idea in the middle and then draw lines from this to other elements of the idea. By that I mean different things I would have to do or think about, organise or book to make this idea happen. I get every part of the idea out onto the paper so there is nothing left in my head. This helps to make the idea happen so much more easily and helps me see if it's actually going to be worth it.*

Journalling: *This is similar to the above but you just write your thoughts down in any way that feels right and gets them out. Often this makes sense and is more of a story/diary and it may be just jumbled up words. It's a great way to get your thoughts out and your emotions and feelings too.*

Tapping/Emotional Freedom Technique (EFT):
Tapping helped me so very much with my stress and anxiety and a whole heap more. It's simple and empowering (as you don't need to see a professional to use it) and it really does work. You tap on meridian points on the body and say exactly what is bothering you (unedited). As you speak your truth about things, it releases mental and physical blockages throughout the body. So it's not only amazing for mental and physical health but it's also a great way to get all your anxiety or stressful thoughts out. Check out Chapter 33 at the end of this book for more information on this technique if it's new to you.

I have noticed that many people who are are recovered or very nearly recovered, really struggle with having too many things to think about when they start doing more (especially going out into the big wide world again). Finding a way to get it all out of your head so you don't find yourself going backwards with your health is very important. So, if you are in this place in your recovery, I urge you to either seriously think about and do one or all of the above regularly or find another way that suits you to get those pesky thoughts out before they create a big-ass-mind-mess for you.

CHAPTER 13
SENSITIVITIES

E veryone I have met with CFS has sensitivities. Not everyone has the same sensitivities but there are some basic ones that at least when we are in very bad/low periods of CFS come and bite most of us on the bum.

Having sensitivities to light, noise, smells, foods and chemicals is common with CFS. These may come and go or be around most of the time, but they are certainly worse when we feel at our most poorly with CFS.

This is because our nervous system in these times is so over-stimulated, it simply cannot cope with anything more.

These are the times when our mind has been in overdrive, worrying, analysing, comparing, regretting, etc. We are really struggling with life and in the fight-or-flight response. Then comes some additional noise, a smell, it gets bright outside, or someone cleans something with bleach, or you eat a tiny bit of cheese (that you were fine with yesterday or last week). This is when the body says enough! Enough of all these stimuli, all this stuff, all these expectations, I cannot heal like this, I need peace.

You go and lay in a dark room, away from all the stimuli, apart from one. That one is your mind. You probably feel a bit better being in that dark, quiet room for a bit; it's less stimulating for sure, but because there is nothing you can do in that moment, your mind starts to wander, giving you a hard time for not being better, not being able to do nice things, be like "normal" people etc.

This is the optimum time to do some of the things laid out in this book, like being really present in your moment, feeling what's there, making friends with your thoughts, embracing your emotions etc. Because if you can come down to a less conflicted place in your mind now, then this over-stimulation you feel will go away, fast.

The more time you can hang out in the less conflicted place, the more healing you can do. The body is stronger and more able to heal when it is not fighting with its mind. When it must fight with the mind as well as the rest of the planet, it becomes easily drained, over-stimulated and then sensitive to all of it.

Sensitivities are no doubt improved if we can remove the things triggering them from our surroundings, like avoiding wheat in our diet, not using toxic washing powers, remembering to wear sunglasses etc. However, that does not solve the reason the sensitivities exist in the first place. To do that, we must find peace in our minds.

CHAPTER 14
PAIN

We all have pain for many different reasons, even when suffering with CFS this is the case. The reasons for your pain will be different to those of the next person with CFS, and the one after that. I cannot "fix" all your aches and pains for you. However, I can tell you what makes them all a lot worse...

The pesky mind again!

No matter what pain you have going on in the body, the mind will make it worse for you, if you let it. As soon as you start to stress or over-think, this will trigger the nervous system which will in turn make your pain symptoms worse.

When we focus on the pain itself (which I know is hard not to do) we make our symptoms worse. So, if possible, it's good not to label the pain as "bad" and "overwhelming" etc., but to try to breathe through it and know it is there for a reason – not because your body is broken but there is a lesson in this madness somewhere.

I suffered most of my life with really intense headaches, and for part of my life, it was one long twelve-year headache that never went away. I tried everything there was to try: some things helped a little, like acupuncture, and at one point when I was younger, reflexology made my headaches go away completely for a couple of years. However, they just kept coming back.

Then one day I realised the head pain, when it was really bad, meant I could not focus on the mental pain I was going through. So, I started to look at the onset of a headache as an invitation to address my mental pain, and the physical pain started to go away. I rarely get headaches now, but when I do, it's always because I have been thinking too much, and when I address this, the head pains start to fade again.

Most physical issues are invitations to address mental stuff going on for us. They won't always make the physical stuff go away, but they almost always lessen the physical pain-load.

Often pain is a protector (remember our bodies are always trying to protect us). So, ask yourself when the pain comes on, what could this be protecting you from? A person, a memory, an event, a thought? Explore that, do your best not to add to your pain with conflict, and see what it's inviting you to explore and be able to resolve or heal.

CHAPTER 15

HEALTH ANXIETY

I think most of us can agree we are at least suffering from low-level but persistent anxieties or just simple, plain old over-thinking.

This is how many people get chronically fatigued. The mind is constantly on the go thinking, analysing and second-guessing. We feel tired but wired. Little things seem like big things but also, we often pride ourselves on how much we are managing to do and how good we are at multi-tasking. Until it all gets too much and we find ourselves with something like CFS.

Well, this same level of over-thinking we had before the CFS doesn't go away, in fact It often gets even worse once we get ill. Then we have the illness to think about, worry about, research, fix, contend with. And because we are not well enough to distract ourselves with much else, it usually becomes our main focus which leads to more anxiety, stress and over-thinking: How can this be happening to me? Why is this happening to me? What did I do wrong?

How do I fix it? How fast can I fix it? How do I find the time to fix it? Is it even fix-able?

If we knew it was just a common cold and would be gone in a week or two, then that would not be so bad, but we've been told it's a long-term thing and we can't do long-term things because we've got lives to lead and things to do.

I guess in a way, much of this book is about health anxiety because it's about reducing our daily conflict to create, not only a healing state, but one where we can function again in that crazy-ass-world.

I have seen it time and again and experienced it myself: the same anxieties that were part of our illness presenting itself in the first place are also what keep us stuck for a while too. To start with it's good, because we focus on getting well and how to do it, but it very easily spirals into a very unhelpful place because we start doing a million different things at once to regain health. We start stressing about how we do things, when we do them, schedules, pacing, toxins, foods, chemicals, relationships – anything we think is triggering our ill health in any way becomes a serious issue for us. What we don't seem to notice is that stressing about all these things is the actual issue itself most of the time, and often not the original thing we were worried about.

Yes, we should all be less toxic in body and home because toxins do add to our health issues, however we should not be trying to be less toxic at the expense of our mental health, because that has a bigger detrimental effect on our wellbeing than many other physical things we are doing.

So, if you are finding yourself doing any of the following, then I invite you to take a breath and ask yourself, "How can I do these things in a less conflicted way?"

➢ Worrying about everything I am eating

➢ Worrying about eating too much/not enough

➢ Worrying about the toxins in my cosmetics

➢ Worrying about the toxins in my home

➢ Worrying about the toxins outside

➢ Worrying about my toxic partner/friend/family member

➢ Worrying about this pain/ache/itch/symptom

➢ Worrying about sleep

➢ Worrying about anything else health-related daily

It is OK to have these concerns, but when they are happening all day long about all sorts of things, you are creating and adding to your mental toxic load, which in turn is triggering the nervous system and making all your physical symptoms much worse too.

Yes, becoming healthy can become consuming, however if you allow it to take a hold where it becomes a health anxiety, then all those good things you are doing for yourself are only half as effective as if you were doing them in a less conflicted and more healing head space.

Remember this question and refer to it daily or even hourly (ha): "How can I do this in a less conflicted way?"

Conflict causes stress and stress fuels the symptoms you are already anxious about.

CHAPTER 16
MOVING FROM HEAD TO HEART

One of the things that helped my mental health more than almost anything else was recognising when I was feeling overwhelmed, stuck, alone, unfocused or sh#tty. I was lost in my head and was not at all in my heart.

Being stuck in our heads makes us over-think things, get anxious, stressed and depressed. This then adds to the heavy load we are already carrying and triggers that nervous system response.

However, when we notice we have been lost in our own crazy brain and its thoughts again, rather than giving ourselves a hard time for being human and feeling mentally rubbish for a while, we should view this lostness as an invitation to return to our heart. When we are born and for the first few years of our life, we are heart-based creatures. We do not care what we look like, sound like, act like, dress like or what shape our body is. We love life. However, we are soon told to behave, be quiet and conform and we learn to be head-centred rather than heart-centred.

So, what we are doing when moving from head to heart is re-learning something that was just instinctive in us when we were small. It takes time to get back into a habit of being more heart-centred – I mean, we have been doing the exact opposite for most of our lives. I recommend setting reminders in your phone or putting up Post-it notes or using your Thriving Guide (more about this in Chapter 35 of this book) to remind yourself to move from head to heart.

Eventually it's just second nature and you will notice when you are back in your head rather than your heart.

Not only does our crazy brain not behave quite so crazy when we hang out more in our hearts, but this is also where we are more creative, flowing, abundant, happy and healthy too.

There are some simple ways to be more heart-centred and these include:

➢ Doing heart-centred guided meditations

➢ Simply placing your hand on your heart and drawing your awareness down to that spot and breathing in and out of this place. The HeartMath Institute in the United States has completed research on this and has said that the body produces "happy" hormones whenever you place your hand on your heart (so that's kinda cool!)

➢ Being out in nature and really present in your moments whilst there

> ➤ Hugging someone (and apparently this is even better if heart to heart)

I recommend you do at least some of these every day and make yourself a vow to be as heart-centred as possible for one month and see the impact it has on your mental health, relationships, creativity and more.

I have some short heart-centred guided meditations on my YouTube channel: http://faithcanter.com/videos/ that may assist with this.

General rule of thumb: If you are feeling s#itty, you are stuck in your head, so move your awareness to your heart and enjoy the ease and peace of hanging out there for a while.

Oh, and don't get me wrong. Our heads aren't bad, and they definitely need to be in charge when we are sorting and doing things, but much of the time they are being so influenced by our need to fit in with the rest of society, our past and our ego, that they actually make us deeply unhappy and unwell instead.

CHAPTER 17

BE MINDFUL OF YOUR MOMENTS

Be mindful of your moment! Sounds simple, right? Well it is, but it's the remembering that isn't always so simple (the Thriving Guide mentioned in Chapter 35 of this book will help with this part though).

When you are in overwhelm, everything is too much, you are too sensitive, too stimulated, everything's loud, bright, too intense – then come right back to the moment, to what is right in front of you. I do not mean you need to start writing a gratitude journal or counting your blessings or anything even as complicated as that (although this is good too). I mean that wherever you are right now, stop... and feel the moment.

Feel like a child would feel for the first time when they are exploring something new. Because you too are also exploring something new, something you never noticed before or not properly or for a long time. Touch the fabric of the duvet, or the sofa or the carpet, feel it, wherever you are right now. Feel its texture, softness, folds, roughness, ridges. Be present with the experience of just feeling, just being present in this moment with this fabric. Feel around you and do the same with wherever your hands or feet wander to. Breathe. Be. Experience.

The more you do this, the easier it will become and then you will find yourself doing it even without trying too. You will start experiencing more of your surroundings rather than feeling so caged in by them, and you will appreciate more of what is around you. Most importantly, you'll come out of the overwhelm quicker and happier.

Being mindful of our moments allows us to be in a less conflicted, more healing place more frequently, and stops the crazy brain from making us crazier, unhealthier and unhappier.

Remember: It's quality, not quantity!

CHAPTER 18

LET'S STOP MAKING EVERY NEW ACHE, PAIN OR ITCH A NEW SYMPTOM

Every single ache, pain, itch, strange feeling or new symptom does not have to be CFS getting worse, unless you make it that way.

What do I mean by this?

I mean that when you have been ill for a long time, you are in a place of heightened awareness of your body and you notice everything happening to it, more than people without CFS do. This can be good because you don't overdo things or pushyourself as much as you may have done before, however it's also not helpful too. This is because you start to label everything that's happening as a new strange symptom so you must be getting worse.

The thing is, every single person on this planet has strange aches, pains, itches and weirdnesses happening in their body from time to time. But mostly these are just brushed off as having slept awkwardly, overexerting something or just something random that's bound to go away soon enough.

What starts to happen more often than not with CFS sufferers is that the new ache, pain or itch triggers the nervous system response because it starts the mind worrying about what it is, is it worse, how long have I had this, etc? This, in turn, makes us feel worse mentally and physically and then, not only do we have this "new symptom" to worry about, but we do feel worse (so there we go, we are getting worse, we were right).

Is would be really, really, really good to remember (and add to the Thriving Guide – more about this in Chapter 35 of this book) that not every new ache, pain, itch or strange feeling is a new symptom of our CFS getting worse. Sometimes, just like non-CFS sufferers, we get strange things happening for short periods of time in our body, just randomly.

When we don't focus on these things and make them into something bad, we don't trigger the nervous system and make ourselves feel mentally and physically worse, and we also don't reinforce the thing we are worried about and thus make it into "a thing".

The mind cannot tell the difference between imagining something and the real thing, hence we have panic attacks and anxiety about things that have not happened or may not ever happen, because our thoughts make our mind believe that it is happening. This is also why visualisation (more about this later too) is super-powerful for working towards full health, because it helps to focus the mind on what we do want instead of what we do not.

Not everything going on in your body is your body getting worse (write that down!)

CHAPTER 19

ALLOW YOUR BODY TO RELEASE

Allowing your body to "release" sounds simple but it also seems it's one of the things we may struggle with the most.

Your body is super-intelligent and knows what to do to heal itself. Unfortunately, the mind gets in the way and thinks it knows better. Then we add to that further and we start to believe other people know better than our own body does, and we start to do what they tell us to do.

We have gradually been taught not to trust our own bodies and our own ability to heal and instead, to look outside for what is within.

No doubt before you got CFS, there were many times when your body wanted you to stop, rest or slow down. You may have kept getting ill or put your back out or found yourself saying you just needed to rest or get a better night's sleep. These are not random concerns, these are your body saying, please, please will you rest. But we don't listen, so the body whispers louder and we have more of these thoughts and feelings and generally become more run down, poorly and tired.

The thing is, your body doesn't hold it against you, it will continue to assist your healing, you just need to learn to let it do its thing and things will be easier for it and you.

One of the things your body is constantly doing its best to do is release. It wants to release toxins and traumas. It does not want to hold on to them, forever in their grip, it wants them gone so it can function better.

The mind is the same, it wants to release toxic thoughts and traumas in the same way the body wants to, for example, the body would prefer to sweat a lot of toxins out, but we don't like to smell, so we put anti-perspirants on. The body has to find other ways. It would really like to remove the toxins through urine too, but you don't drink enough because you are busy, or you don't like urinating all the time.

So physically you can see the body is doing its thing, even when you fight against it, but mentally this is happening too.

It's likely that either before being diagnosed with CFS or soon after, you may have had times of intense yawning, crying, shaking, sweating or sickness. This is the body trying to release and let go of trauma (and also purge itself of toxins). But we don't like the feeling of these things happening in our body so what we do is we try to stop it. We take anti-sickness medication, sedatives and other pills, potions and lotions to prevent the body from doing something that it wants and needs to do.

If you are even slightly suspicious that you are toxic or suffering from trauma, then I invite you to listen to what you body is trying to do to release this, and just let it go ahead and do it. But remember, it's unlikely to be over quickly because it's got a lifetime of these sorts of things to release. The releasing could be days of sickness, weeks of yawning or months of shaking or crying. Let it flow! Let your body release it. These things are not bad, they are very good in fact. How else do you expect your body to release trauma and toxins if not physically?

Of course, if you are sick for a prolonged period of time, consult your doctor, but short periods of sickness are a great release for us both mentally and physically.

Think about how the animal kingdom deals with such things. After a deer escapes from a lion, it does not need to go and have therapy for ten years because of the trauma. It shakes constantly for a while and releases that trauma and then gets on with its life. Our bodies try to do the same. When we go into shock we shake, but then the people around us usually try to help us to stop shaking, thinking it's bad for us, when in fact it's the opposite.

Body tremors and restless legs are also apparently the body trying to release trauma. So let it happen, let it be, and, if anything, encourage it, shake some more. You could see someone trained in Total Release Experience (TRE), breathwork or some other form of trauma release therapy.

CHAPTER 20
WHAT IS THIS AN INVITATION TO RESOLVE?

J ust a quick note on those triggers and why they could really be there.

When we feel triggered by something or someone, rather than start blaming anyone and everyone involved, (including ourselves), a great new habit I invite you to form and add to your Thriving Guide (more about this in Chapter 35 of this book) is to ask yourself the following question:

"What is this an invitation to explore or change in order to resolve and heal?"

For instance, when we are triggered by someone rejecting us or hurting us etc:

Rejection: *Why is this happening? Is it because we have been rejecting ourselves? We don't feel good enough? We are being redirected because this thing or person isn't for us? What is the real reason it hurts? What can we learn from this? How can we grow from this? What can we let go of? What should we explore resolving within us? How can we* give ourselves this instead? What is this inviting me to change?

Hurt: Why is this hurting? What old habit or pattern of thinking has this triggered? Have I been doing this to myself? Am I expecting someone else to treat me right when I do not treat myself right? Am I attached to this person? How can I let go of this hurt? What is this inviting me to change?

When we look for the learnings in the things that trigger us or cause us pain, then they have less power over us next time and we grow through our discomfort too. It's all here for a reason and that reason isn't to make us feel more rubbish!

CHAPTER 21

LET'S NOT BE VICTIMS

Some of you may find this topic triggers you – I know it was for me to start with. However, it's a topic I feel is important to address and if you do find yourself triggered by it, then it's one that I invite you to explore more of too, because we are generally not triggered if all is well.

In our society, we gain something from being a victim. We often get attention, love, support, companionship, thoughts, kind words and assistance.

Many of us have been abused and used in our early years and it makes us feel (rightly so) a victim. It's true – we were a victim. We were treated badly. However, it's not healthy to keep allowing ourselves to dwell in that victim mentality. As mentioned earlier in this book, this means the abuser/user/person has effectively "won" – they still have power or control over us.

The other reason why it's not healthy for us is because it becomes a means to get the things we feel are missing, like support, love, attention.

When we are chronically ill, of course we cannot help but feel a victim; life sucks, and sometime because of it we do get those things we are lacking, and it does really help us.

The problem is when it becomes our "label" or what identifies us. When we see ourselves as a victim of life due to this illness, others see this in us too.

This is not healthy because although it may feel like it sometimes, we don't have to be a victim. Being a victim keeps us stuck because those thoughts of "poor me", "what did I do to deserve this?" or "I must have done something really bad in a previous life," trigger that nervous system response again and keep us stuck exactly where we are. Thought like this also get you nowhere but going around in circles again.

If we can recognise that things do suck at the moment but then accept that this is part of the illness, we can learn how to live in a less conflicted way. Then we can feel these feelings, but hopefully not get so deeply sucked under by them. Try not to rely on others for support, love and attention and if we do get that attention, it's because they willingly want to give it and not because they feel sorry for us. Being a victim of whatever life throws at you just isn't helpful for making change. However, if we see that we have been doing this, be OK with the fact that we lost our way for a bit because we are human and chronically ill. Then see what this feeling is inviting us to explore within ourselves so that we can move on from it, rather than feeling crushed by this illness and life in general – don't let these thoughts keep us stuck right where we don't want to be.

CHAPTER 22
SECONDARY GAINS

S econdary gains is another one of those topics that you may find a bit triggering, I know I certainly did.

It's hard to believe we may actually be gaining something from our illness and that this could possibly be what is keeping us stuck at a subconscious level.

When I finally decided I was going to work on my potential secondary gains, I did feel some big shifts happen and I have seen this happen in others too.

Secondary gains are things that we gain from being ill. So, this could be things like not having to go to work/ leaving our really horrible job/not having to attend family or social gatherings/people doing things for us/support/ assistance/we have a good excuse to leave things early that we don't like/etc.

When you think about how your illness may work in your favour, what comes to mind?

It may be that it starts an argument in your mind. What I mean by this is, you may feel sometimes it's great that you don't have to work in that super-stressful and horrible place any more, but then at other times, you might really, really want the opportunity/health/energy to be able to work again – this is true for many.

Just because you gain from your illness in some way, it doesn't mean you don't wish for things to be different. No one wants to be ill and stuck at home, but there are some things that being ill protects us from – like horrible people/ jobs and having to sort out banking/insurance/important and stressful stuff which our partner, family member or carer has done for us up until now.

If you know deep down that sometimes, in a tiny way, your illness works in your favour, then I invite you to tap (more about this in Chapter 33 of this book) on this and get it cleared. I would invite you to say out loud all the ways your illness is helping you. Then consider all the ways you can give yourself permission to release this assistance and be open to finding new ways of speaking and living your truth, without relying on the illness to support you in any way.

Our subconscious mind is a tricky thing and I am never surprised by how it can screw us over without our even realising it. So, I invite you to spend some time clearing this, maybe even journal about it if you are not ready to tap on it yet, and remove anything at all that may possibly be holding back full health.

And one last thing, I invite you to think about the reasons you give for not doing things. Rather than, "I feel really ill/tired/wired etc. so I cannot do/come/be/stay", try rephrasing it instead like, "It's really not for me/I only have a limited amount of energy at the moment and I would prefer to spend it on something else/that person is draining for me/I just don't want to do this", etc. Speaking our truths is super-empowering and even energising, and allows us to move through things and release other things. If more of us spoke our truths, things would be a lot easier around here.

CHAPTER 23
STOP SEARCHING FOR PURPOSE

I notice that as sufferers start to move along their road to recovery, (and I admit I did this too,) we get fixated on purpose/future/life goals etc. What will I do when I'm well? How will I do it? How will I fund it? What if I do it and it makes me ill again? What if I do it and it's not for me? How do I know what's for me? etc.

This is obviously all causing a stress response, triggering the nervous system and making us feel worse, which is the exact opposite of what we are trying to achieve.

What I noticed with my own recovery and that of everyone else I have been involved with, is that we cannot "think up" a purpose. It will come.

One of the great teachings of CFS is that it shows us a new and healthier way to be "us" in the world and this means whatever we came here to do also.

It will come; whatever we are meant to be will become clear, as soon as we stop trying to focus on it and make it happen.

My clients and members of my membership group hear me say time and time again, "Follow your heart." Make more time for hanging out in the heart, with guided heart meditations, simply putting your hand on your heart and bringing you awareness there or being really present in nature (or your garden), letting go of the nonsense of the brain trying to "fix, change and improve" everything. When we are more heart-centred, we are more creative - fact!

You cannot think up your purpose; you'll feel it instead though, when you stop trying to figure it out.

What do you enjoy doing? Do that. While you have the time and the little bits of energy here and there, do things that feel good to do. Sit in nature, write poetry/songs/blogs, or study gardening/embroidery/mechanics/whatever interests you. Follow your fun and see where things flow to. Your purpose will become clear when you remain open to exploring what lights you up.

I have encouraged some clients who were already writers in some way to get all their frustrations about the illness out in words somehow. It's been incredibly healing for them and allows others to see they are not alone and there are other people out there who understand how they feel.

Creativity in any form at all is deeply healing for us and will, in some way, lead to whatever is next for us on our path, because it keeps us open and exploring who we are and how we fit into this crazy-ass-world.

CHAPTER 24

WHEN I AM WELL I WILL DO THESE THINGS...

It's so easy to focus on what we cannot do when we have been unwell for a long time. But all this does for us is make us upset, frustrated and depressed. This, in turn, makes all our symptoms worse and leaves us less likely to be able to do much else.

It's good to have a mantra or something like this:

"When I am well I will do these things, but for now I will focus my attention on what I can do right now to allow this to happen in the future."

So, yes, you may not be able to walk to the shop, sort the laundry or go out with friends now. But, instead of getting upset about this, ask yourself what you can do right now that would assist these things to happen for you in the future?

It may be that you can visualise these things happening now. Or you have a good old tap (more about this in Chapter 33 of this book) to release all the frustrations and upsets. Or you go and ground yourself in the garden, taking some deep cleansing breaths and feeling more centred and in a place to be able to heal once more. Or you go and eat something nourishing and energising for you.

We can't help getting upset by this restricted life, so if you lose your way and find yourself doing that, then let it out, let it flow and let it go. But, sometimes just remembering that all these negative emotions are fuel for the very things we do not want is enough to remind you that you can do something more healing with your time right now and go do that instead.

I invite you to consider adding this to your Thriving Guide (details in Chapter 35 of this book), as a reminder that you can choose to fuel health or fuel fear.

CHAPTER 25

THE TWO MOST IMPORTANT FACTORS

It is my belief that the two most important factors to gaining freedom from CFS and many long-term illnesses are to focus on both our mental health and our digestive health and to do these two things at the same time.

Our mental health effects our digestive health, so if you are just trying to heal your digestive system without working with your mind, you will only get so far and probably find you will continue to have digestive flare-ups.

Your digestive health affects your mental health, because around 70% of your serotonin (known as the "happy hormone") is produced in your gut, so if you try to address just your mental health without addressing your digestive health, you'll only get so far this way too.

Working with both at the same time is a perfect union for freedom from ill health.

Most of this book is giving you ways to make friends with your thoughts and live in a less conflicted and more healing state, but at this point, I want to tackle how to address any unhealthy digestive system too.

Everyone I have met with CFS and most long-term health conditions has an imbalance in the digestive system. This often means there are yeast and parasite issues, food intolerances, bloating, poor nutrient absorption and general IBS type symptoms.

Although avoiding trigger foods and stress helps, it does not address the imbalance. To do this I invite you to consider consuming fermented foods and drinks (kombucha, kefir, sauerkraut and kimchi etc). I don't mean pickled foods and drinks (or beer, ha!) I mean lacto-fermented (with salt and water) foods. This not only preserves all the goodness from the fruits and vegetables used but creates a super-strong probiotic food or drink. There are many more probiotics in these foods and drinks than in most probiotics tablets or drinks you can buy from a pharmacy.

These foods and drinks help to address the imbalance created by long-term illness, medications, burning the candle at both ends, stress and eating badly that has built up over our lifetime.

Please start small though, if you have a serious imbalance, the fermented foods and drinks will make you detox, (ie: run off to the toilet frequently!) It's not that you are now intolerant to these too, it's that your imbalance is so bad, you only need a teeny tiny amount of these foods and drinks to start with, and then you very slowly build up.

These foods and drinks are very simple to make and last many months so when you are feeling up to it, make up a big batch that will last months, or ask a family member or friend to do this as a birthday gift or something like that. You can buy these products from health food shops too, but it works out quite expensive as they must be the unpasteurised versions, not the pasteurised ones (with little goodness in) that you'll pick up in a supermarket.

Once you have got used to consuming regular amounts of fermented foods and drinks, I would invite you to look into doing a yeast and parasite cleanse. Almost everyone I meet, no matter if they are long-term ill or not, has a yeast and parasite issue. A yeast and parasite overgrowth shows itself in much the same way as CFS does - digestive issues, fatigue, brain fog, memory issues, skin complaints and general aches. So, this overgrowth is making all your symptoms worse.

Doing a yeast and parasite cleanse is like a reboot for the body, as it affects most of our internal systems. It's a great way to bring yourself back into balance but also allows the body to start to function more efficiently and usually means that more energy, better mood, happier hormones and clearer thinking occur too.

A cleanse like this is quite intense and that is why I am recommending you start with a small amount of fermented foods and drinks first to help your body and mind get into a stronger place for beginning a cleanse.

You can find details of cleanses like this all over the internet or you can check out my book Cleanse – A Holistic Detox Program For Mind, Body & Soul. The whole book is dedicated to this cleanse but not only this, it takes you through ways to support your cleanse with things for your mind, (tapping, meditation etc.), and ways to support the body while it is releasing the yeasts, parasites and toxins. It also has lots of recipes within it to inspire you and heaps of supporting videos to watch alongside doing the cleanse online.

Remember: when you work with mind and digestive system together, you will have a bigger positive impact on your health than working with either separately because they are both so intertwined.

Oh, and there are heaps of fermenting recipes to inspire you on my website too!

CHAPTER 26

FOLLOWING AN ADRENALLY SUPPORTIVE LIFESTYLE

One of the greatest things you, or anyone for that matter, can do for your health if you are in the least bit stressed, anxious, depressed or an overthinker, is to create an adrenally supportive lifestyle.

It is my belief that most people, before being diagnosed with CFS have had adrenal fatigue (extreme exhaustion and mental impairment bought on by chronic stress and/or infection) for many years. So, if we assist the underlying adrenal fatigue, then we address the CFS. It's also a great thing to remember once you are free from CFS and are perhaps going through a stressful period in your life.

Many people out there are suffering from some level of adrenal fatigue, so your family and friends may want to get involved or consider what I share here. You'll know if you or someone else is suffering from adrenal fatigue (tests are usually not very accurate) because you will notice that any degree of stress affects your mental and physical health very badly and you rarely feel better, even after a good rest.

Physically, the best way to support the adrenals is to reduce your stress levels, (using all the techniques in this book), and also in a few other ways too. For instance, we are all told exercise is good for us, but when you become obsessed with it or are pushing harder and harder all the time despite feeling tired and drained already, then this stresses the adrenal system rather than helping them. Training for long runs or tackling assault courses etc. may be fun, but if you are already in a stressed place mentally, this extra physical stress can push you over the edge. (I have often heard of this happening in people's stories about where they felt their CFS began).

The same goes for overworking. If you are already feeling the pull of exhaustion, then working harder, longer or more is going to add to the stress on the adrenals. Hence, why when you have a little bit of energy and you decide to do a million things to make up for all you could not do in the last week or two, you add mental and physical stress to your adrenals (plus your body isn't that fit at the moment either, so it becomes more tired more quickly).

The dietary changes are usually a bit harder for people because, well, you have no energy for most physical things once you are ill anyway, and you may also resort to using things like caffeine and sugars for an energy boost when you have CFS.

The thing is, that anything that spikes your blood sugars (giving you a bit of an extra energy boost or fix) is affecting the proper function of your adrenals and is also going to leave you always searching for the next fix.

What we want to do to support the adrenals through diet is reduce the things that spike the blood sugars and consume more things that help to keep our blood sugar levels balanced. Firstly, it's better to eat a little every three or four hours than wait for a big meal at dinner time. This helps maintain balance. The next most important thing is to reduce or remove the following food items from your diet:

➢ Processed sugars

➢ High sugar fruits (banana, pineapple, papaya, mango and grapes)

➢ White carbohydrates (white potatoes, white rice, pasta, flours and breads)

➢ Caffeine in any form (even green teas)

➢ Alcohol

Replace these with as much sweet potato, brown/red/black rice, quinoa, millet, vegetables (especially leafy greens) and all other fruits (especially berries), fats, oils, seeds and nuts as you like.

Even though I had a fairly healthy diet before, I was still heavily reliant on white carbs and "free-from" foods (which are mostly all full of sugars and crap) and if I had to go out for something, I'd have lemonade or a green tea to keep me going. But this is just borrowed energy and is another of the reasons we often crash. Together with the stress factor and the fact we are not that fit now, there is also the fact that we have topped up our non-existent energy reserve with sugars and caffeine to make it through. These things may help us feel better temporarily but long-term, they are very detrimental to our health.

It was tricky for me to give up white potatoes and rice to start with as these are easy, yummy, comfort foods. However, after a short while, I found I preferred brown rice and sweet potato wedges (they are also more nutrient dense). And I still eat more of these than I do white carbo-hydrates to this day.

Just try to replace one thing a week if it all sounds a bit too much, and notice how you feel after you do consume something that spikes the blood sugar levels. I bet to start with you feel great, but as the come-down arrives, are you searching for another hit to bring you back up again and do you feel even more exhausted and even depressed from it?

Feel into what these foods and drinks are really doing to you mentally and physically and try to replace or reduce them where you can: your adrenal system and thus your mental and physical health will thank you for it.

There are also herbs and supplements that assist the body with adrenal fatigue, but they won't help on their own, you do need to address the triggers as mentioned above.

CHAPTER 27
LYMPHATIC SUPPORT

Most people's lymphatic system is struggling these days. This includes people without chronic illnesses too. There are just too many toxins that we are taking on board every single day that overload the system designed to eliminate these things.

However, it is possible to support the lymphatic system in its bid to remove the toxins already on board and those we'll continue to take on board daily too.

You'll see a lot of people in the CFS community talking about supporting the lymphatic system because this really is important in assisting us to reduce the toxic load of the body.

A certain amount of gentle exercise can help for starters. Things like getting a mini trampoline or an exercise ball and bouncing your whole body up and down, or if you are unable to do this, then just bouncing your feet and legs up and down. This helps stimulate the lymphatic system into action, but sometimes even this can be a struggle if you are feeling particularly weak.

However, you can do a thing called body-brushing, and I invite you and everyone else you know to do this daily where possible. Body-brushing alone (without changing diet or anything else) can cause detox symptoms as it starts to support the body in removing the toxins it's been holding on to. This shows you how powerful a tool this is. It's just softly brushing the skin to stimulate the lympathic system to remove toxins and and the build-up of lactic acid in the muscles.   There are CFS treatments out there that focus almost solely on supporting the lymphatic system which appear to have helped CFS sufferers recover.

The one thing I would say is, if you feel you may be super-toxic, then take it slowly and just do a bit each day, because going through a heavy detox whilst having CFS can be intense.

You can buy a brush for this or, like me, you can just use your hands. You brush up your feet, legs, abdomen and breasts, (this is very important so the toxins don't get stuck here), and your forearms up towards the area just above your breasts. Then you brush down down your face and neck to the same area on the chest. Do this for ten minutes each day. If this is too much for you, then just do part of this each time and break it up through out your day.

When you apply creams, potions or lotions or dry your-self after a bath or shower, do your best to remember to always dry upwards. It may seem a little strange to start with, but if you consciously do it for a while then eventu-ally is becomes second nature.

I have a video about this on my YouTube channel: http://faithcanter.com/videos/ if you want to see how it's done. It certainly reduced some of my muscle aches and pains once I started doing it regularly and anyway, if we can get a few more toxins eliminated, we help our bodies to function in a more optimal and healing manner.

CHAPTER 28

BREATH & POSTURE

I wanted to touch on something so simple, yet very over-looked. And I don't just mean for people with CFS but for most of the population of the world.

Most people are not breathing very effectively, and their posture is, well, shocking. This has an impact on people without chronic illness, but even more so for those with.

Without good posture, it is much harder for us to breathe optimally, so the first thing I invite you to become aware of is how you are sitting, standing and lying. Are you crunched over or slouched off to the side? Not only is this not good for your bones and muscles but it makes your organs struggle to do what they need to do for a healthy body. But the thing is here, it's making it harder for your lungs to inflate properly and then circulate that oxygen around the body.

Often, people suffering with CFS are not getting enough oxygen into their system, hence why many sufferers in the UK are offered oxygen therapy from the NHS. So, anything we can do to assist the flow of oxygen in our bodies is helping us.

Where possible try not to slouch, crunch and crush your body too much and for too long, making sure, where possible, that your posture is one of support and flow and thus more oxygen moves around the body, allowing the body to function at a more optimal level.

The other thing to do is to breathe in the most optimum way possible for better oxygen flow. Start the day with some breathing techniques, or do them when you meditate or are waiting for the kettle to boil, whatever feels right. Try to breathe everything (all the stale air) out of the lungs a few times and breathe in full lung-fulls of breath too. By doing this, you let go of stale air and toxins that hide out in the bottom of the lungs, and you receive back much more oxygen for a much happier and healthier body too.

Also, try to do some belly breathing at the same time or some other time during the day. This means when you breathe in, push your belly out and when you breathe out, you draw your belly in. It feels very strange to start with but you soon get the hang of it.

If breathing in and out fully is an issue for you, then breathe to where it feels comfortable, or just do the full emptying of your lungs and don't focus so much on the full breaths in for now.

CHAPTER 29
ELECTROMAGNETIC STRESS

With this technological age come new technological illnesses. Electromagnetic stress (EMS) is the subtle, or not so subtle, effect of stray or chaotic electrical and magnetic fields on the human body. All electrical appliances givs off electrical and magnetic fields when plugged in. We are also exposed to these fields when radio or microwave signals are received or emitted. These electromagnetic fields (EMF), much like our own body fields, vibrate constantly. When they meet the human body field, they can disrupt cell structures, our immune, nervous and endocrine system responses, and increase the risk of tumour formation. We spend so much time around electrical appliances and so little time in nature that more and more people are finding they are suffering from some form of EMS.

The common symptoms of EMS (problems concentrating, anxiety, depression, aggression, irritability, insomnia and general sleep problems, dizziness, fatigue, nausea, respiratory issues, itching, joint and muscle pain, persistent detox symptoms, jitters, eyesight issues, not feeling grounded, memory loss and brain fog) are the same as many of the common symptoms of CFS. And not only that, but you are much more suspectable to EMS when you have CFS, so it has the potential to make many of your symptoms much worse than they already are.

Here are some of my top tips for lessening the EMS load:

➤ Remove as many electrical appliances from your bedroom as possible, especially phones, laptops, tablets and TVs - actually, anything that is receiving or emitting signals of any sort.

➤ Bin the electric blanket; these are possibly one of the worst items for increasing electromagnetic stress because they are so close to us for so many hours at a time.

➤ Electric clocks, clock radios and baby monitors should be at least one metre away from you.

➤ Switch off as many appliances at night as possible, and when you are not using them.

➤ Do away with your microwave. Not only do microwaves break down most of the nutrients in your food, they are also a big source of electromagnetic stress.

➤ Cordless landline phones are just as bad as mobile phones, so if you need to use these, then try to store them as far away from your body as possible when not in use.

> Unplug yourself. By this I mean spend some time away from all appliances, get out in nature if you can.

> Purchase a grounding mat or blanket for your bed. When you are sleeping, you will be grounding yourself. These earth through the normal plug sockets in your home. You can also pick up smaller ones to place on or under your desk to help when you are surrounded by office equipment.

> Try to avoid wearing rubber-soled shoes and slippers as much as possible, as you are unable to ground/earth through these. You can actually buy earthing shoes, slippers and sandals these days, which help you earth as you are walking.

> Practice grounding meditations and visualisations.

> Consider wearing and/or placing any of the following crystals next to your bed or desk to help minimise the effects of electromagnetic stress: Smoky Quartz, Hematite, Tourmalated Quartz, Black Tourmaline, Amazonite, Sodalite and Unakite.

> Purchase a bio-band, a bio-tag, a grounding egg, earthing necklace or one of the other many grounding items you can carry around on your person all the time to help deflect the harmful effects of electromagnetic stress.

> Consider having amalgam fillings removed. They can make the effects of this type of stress even

worse, because the metals in your mouth attract electromagnetic waves.

➤ Drink plenty of fresh, pure water as this has a wonderful grounding effect on the body.

➤ Use a Zapper, this is a little box that not only grounds you but helps eliminate toxins, yeasts and parasites too.

➤ Get grounding, get as much of your skin in contact with nature as you can. Walk or sit barefoot in the garden and hug trees. Twenty minutes a day brings the body back into balance and assists its natural rhythms and functions.

CHAPTER 30
TAKE A REST FROM GETTING WELL

I know this may sound crazy as you are in an enforced "rest" a lot of the time as a CFS sufferer, but taking a rest from getting well should be prescribed regularly to people trying to recover from CFS. Why? Because we make getting well stressful. We are constantly searching for the next thing to make us well, to enhance our health and quality of life in some way, and it's bloody exhausting! In fact, it's insane what we do to ourselves, and how draining we make getting well become.

It's almost essential we take regular rest, or holidays if you like, from getting well. To step back, replenish, reboot and renew. Even getting well takes energy and if we keep giving to this in a stressful way, then this is going to drain us too.

Even when we are too unwell to actively do every tiny little good thing for our health, every minute of every day, we often give ourselves a hard time for not doing enough.

So, if you have been caught in the cycle of trying desperately to get well, to research and try to fund wellness each and every day, take a rest, take a holiday, have today or tomorrow off. Watch some rubbish on TV, read a fun book instead of another book on wellness, stop googling s#@t online, and do whatever you are able to do, just to have some fun or free time and do your best not to give yourself a hard time for it.

The illness will still be there tomorrow, you can start again then and you'll be fresher and maybe even stronger for having taken a day out of trying desperately to get well.

CHAPTER 31
DO WHAT YOU CAN, WHEN YOU CAN

Doing what you can when you can is tricky, because for most people with CFS, the normal way of functioning is boom or bust. By this I mean, we are in "bust mode" when we are not able to do much. Then we feel a bit better, so all of a sudden, to make up for the bust, we move into "boom mode" and do loads whilst we are feeling OK. Then, suddenly, we are in bust again.

I am here to give you permission, again, to listen to your body and do what feels right, but also to stop when it no longer does. It is OK to leave things half done!

In fact, it's essential to leave things half done.

If you do not have the energy to do something to completion, then just do what you can, please don't push on through and then await your reward of a crash.

Washing four dishes from a stack of dishes is still four dishes less to wash the next time. Just having a shower but not washing your hair because you arms ache too much is fine, at least you don't smell anymore;o). Just tidying one drawer when you want to tidy the whole room, is still one drawer sorted.

Do what you can when you can, and don't push on through when you know you are already totally spent! Because, once you are in that rewarded crash from doing too much, no one, not even you will care about the dishes! And, to top it off, it's likely you'll make the crash worse by telling yourself lots of bad things about how you made it happen, and how you are never going to get better, etc.

Nothing matters more than your mental and physical health, no one cares more about the dishes than they do for you. Listen, learn and let it go.

CHAPTER 32

HOW TO TELL WHEN YOU ARE ON YOUR WAY TO RECOVERY

I am often asked how you know if you are close to recovery, or if you are even doing any better than you were, because you still crash. The latter is easy if you keep a journal, or at least are putting your thoughts anywhere else than keeping them in your head. It's easy not to notice the improvements you have made until you look back on where you were. I didn't notice my improvements to start with and when I would crash, I would keep telling myself that I wasn't getting anywhere. My husband, however, would point out how much I was doing now that I could not before, which I could not see because I was in a bad place mentally. So, look back regularly on your notes/social media posts/journals/diaries/writings to see how far you have actually come, to see that you are moving forward, even if it feels like you have not.

As for the actual recovery part, you can tell when you are on your road to recovery when you take less and less time to get over any mental and/or physical exertion.

Things that might have taken you several days to recover from before, start to take just one or two days, then just one sleep and you are OK and so on.

You go from being able to do one or two things a week to being able to do something every other day, then once a day, then two things a day and so on.

It's important to remember that in this time you can easily feel tired or drained or feel a flare-up of your old symptoms and it does not mean you are in a crash or you've overdone it. So please do your best not to feed into these thoughts, but just recognise that you are simply unfit and not strong yet because your body hasn't done a lot for a long time. Being unfit is fine and to be expected. Giving yourself a hard time for this normal body reaction does not help your progress, in fact it does the opposite and can create a crash – the very thing you want to avoid.

If your friend who was well and healthy did not normally do any running but went for a short run around the neighbourhood, they would be tired and need to rest. They might go to bed early or eat a bit more as their body isn't used to it and isn't strong enough for how far they pushed themselves. Remember this in your own recovery: your body is not used to doing much. It's not that you are becoming unwell again - far from it - but your thoughts and fears of becoming unwell again can cause a relapse, because they trigger your nervous system into action again.

Take things easy, be aware of your thoughts and day by day, and week by week, slowly increase your "training" for living a full life again, just like an athlete would train for a big race.

Nourish your body and mind in the correct way: rest, listen, learn, explore, correct and where possible, remain in a place of less conflict and your body will do the rest.

CHAPTER 33

EMOTIONAL FREEDOM TECHNIQUE / TAPPING

One of the most successful things I have tried and which I still use regularly to this day, is Emotional Freedom Technique (EFT) / Tapping. If you have never heard of this, here is a brief overview. EFT was founded by Gary Craig and makes use of acupuncture points (but without the needles!) With the tips of your fingers, you tap on certain points on the body whilst verbalising areas of concern; this releases the blockages created in the body by toxic thoughts. The hold these thoughts have over us is then released and most importantly, patterns associated with these thoughts are broken. It's like a counselling session but without having to open up to someone about your deepest, darkest thoughts.

For it to work most effectively, you take yourself back in your mind to the first time you had the issue or concern and tap on one of the points of your body, focussing your mind on how this made you feel, both physically and emotionally. If you can address the root cause of the concern, then all the other times this has affected you since then will most likely be addressed in this session also. It is an extremely powerful tool and can release a lot of hurt, negative emotions, toxic thoughts and long-standing negative beliefs about yourself and others. This not only has positive psychological benefits, but it helps all sorts of physical issues that were created or exacerbated by these underlying thought patterns. It can help anything from back pain and weight loss to your love life and depression. If you look up EFT / Tapping, you might get confused by all the different types and methods you find. Please don't be put off; you can keep it simple. In fact that's how I teach and use it now and it's super-effective this way as we actually tap on the thoughts and feelings, not what we think we should be tapping on instead.

I won't go into the traditional way of tapping here because you can look that up yourself. I found that although the traditional way is very effective, it can be a little over-complicated at times, (which with CFS can feel overwhelming I know,) and it can get a bit heady and robotic too. What I have since found to be super-effective is what I call "the easy way to tap". This way, we generally just focus on the one tapping point at a time (or more if that feels right to you).

I like to use the "Karate Chop" point, which is the side of the hand with your little finger on; you tap this into the palm of the other hand. This one can be used anywhere, even if you are sat in traffic, which is when many people start to get stressed and agitated. This easy way of tapping is about working on raw emotions in the moment. When we work with our thoughts, feelings and emotions like this, we can have big shifts, quickly, because we are "in it". It's raw, it's true and it's not thinking about what we think we need to tap on, but instead what is already going on for us in our heads. This way, we just tap on our exact thoughts, unedited, swear words 'n all.

I know this can sound kind of backwards to a lot of alternative practices and ideas, because instead of trying to think, say or do something in a positive way, (like positive affirmations), we are doing the opposite. We are voicing or honouring our perceived negative thoughts. For me, this is super-important and powerful. Having spent a lifetime trying to be positive and not understanding why I never succeeded for very long, I can see why. Because I was pushing parts of me away, not honouring the bits than made me, me. If you are saying a million positive things to yourself every day, but on the inside doing the opposite, then you are going to cause yourself a whole load of conflict, stress and anxiety instead.

So, we tap on all the crappy thoughts and feelings and then when we have got those out, we put in some good stuff. But again, we don't go from saying things like "I hate my body and life" to "I love my body and life", because of course, this will cause conflict, unless we really believe it. The better approach here is to use words like "permission" or "open". What I mean by this is, instead of saying, "I love my body and life" (unless you believe it), I would recommend saying, "I am open to loving my body and life" or "I give myself permission to love my body and life". This sends a powerful message to the subconscious mind that maybe you are open to doing just that.

Giving ourselves permission is an important one, especially if we have been ill for a long time. When I was chronically ill with CFS, giving myself permission to be well again seemed to create a big shift in me. I was so used to being ill and its label, that giving myself permission to be something else was big. The positive tapping at the end of the process should incorporate some of the negative stuff you said at the beginning. So, if you said things like "I am broken / incomplete / need fixing / fat / thin / screwed up", then the positive bits at the end could be something like: I am open to not feeling whole / complete / healed / I give myself permission to feel complete / I am open to not feeling like I need fixing / I give myself permission to love my body / I am open to not feeling screwed up, or even, I give myself permission to be ok with feeling screwed up. You can also add in things that resonate all of a sudden that have nothing to do with what you are tapping on.

I have a whole playlist about tapping on my YouTube channel: http://faithcanter.com/videos/ which you can watch for guidance, and some tapping sequences you can follow. Remember: tap on what you are thinking and not what you think you should be tapping on!

CHAPTER 34
VISUALISATION

Visualisation is a super-powerful yet super-simple technique.

I believe part of the reason for this is because when we have been ill long-terms we are actually spending much of our day focusing on (and thus fuelling) all the things wrong with us, so when we visualise, we do the opposite of this, fuelling the things we do want in our body and life instead.

Instead of focusing every day on how unwell, unfit or fat/ thin you are, I would like to invite you to do the opposite. I don't mean think about how you want to be in the future, I mean focus on feeling that way now. This is the "trick" to effective visualisations – imagine it happening to you now, look down and see your body doing it. You are not watching yourself doing it somewhere else, you are doing it in your imagination. Remember I said near the beginning of this book, the subconscious mind doesn't know the difference between fact and fiction so believes the good things you are focusing on are happening and starts to make changes as such. When you look in the mirror, see yourself how you want to be. Start and/or finish all your meditations, quiet times or even sleeps with a short visualisation where you fully embody being everything you are wanting to be now. Feel it, see it, love it, be it with every cell of your being. Smile, feel the sun/wind/rain, feel the clothes and sweat on your body, everything you can imagine about the situation happening to you now, imagine.

When we are focusing on what we don't want every day, we are creating chemical reactions in the mind that reinforce these negative pathways and thus keep us unwell. However, when we spend time focusing on what we do want (rather than how we feel we are right now), these same reactions happen but instead they create positive pathways for change, thus assisting the body to heal.

I can't state how incredibly powerful this simple technique is, it helped me so much with my own recovery from CFS and I know it helps so many others every single day.

Make a pledge with yourself to try it for a month and see what a profound effect it can have on you.

I have some visualisations on my YouTube channel: http://faithcanter.com/videos/ you can do to get you in the swing of things.

CHAPTER 35

THE THRIVING GUIDE

Versions of the Thriving Guide have featured in two of my other books, but with each new edition, this guide evolves.

The reason I started using it myself and with clients is because when we are in a bad headspace, we will convince ourselves that we have tried everything within our power to change it -that we have been eating well, meditating, being grateful and a whole heap of other things. When in fact, if we were honest and not trying to play mind-games with ourselves, we probably haven't. We may have sat down to meditate, but in fact we were simply listing all the crappy things happening at that moment. It's so easy for things to slip and us not to realise why they have. When we are feeling good, we often forget to do all the things we know help us both mentally and physically. Then when we are not so good, stuff starts to build up and we are less prepared for it and before we know it, we are totally consumed by the negativity of whatever is happening to us. Then, every time without fail, we will convince ourselves we have done everything we could be doing to resolve this.

The Thriving Guide is basically a list of all the things that assist us both mentally and physically to feel happy and healthy. It also includes prompts/questions etc. for us to explore when we are losing our way and could easily end up in "the Pits of Despair" as I have lovingly called it over the years.

So, what you need to do (when you're in a good frame of mind) to create such a list is to get a piece of A4 paper and draw two lines down it, to create three columns. At the top of the first column, write "What Nurtures" and at the top of the middle one write "Naughty Notes" and at the top of the last one write "Conscious Change".

Then in the first column, write a list of all the things you know assist your health, happiness and harmony. These may be things you have tried in the past, things like take a bath, meditate, get out in nature, or they may be some of the things from this book that resonate with you.

In the second column, consider ways in which you can get through to your not-so-emotionally-strong self that you may not be doing the things on the first list. Put the list in order of things that work for you and then you can work your way down as and when you need to.

Then, in the last column, write down how you are going to consciously make sure these things start to happen for your health, happiness and harmony.

Add the things from this book that have resonated with you and questions to ask yourself when you are struggling that might help to understand why you feel like you do and what you can do about it, and then refer to this list daily, checking in on it and yourself before things get too out of hand and the crazy brain really takes over.

To keep the price of this book down for all you lovely readers, I decided I was not going to have images and charts etc. in the book. However, you can see how to create your own guide on my YouTube channel: http://faithcanter.com/videos/

Here are some ideas of things to add to your Thriving Guide:

What Nurtures: Am I meditating? – *Naughty Notes – Really Faith? Or are you making shopping lists in your mind? - Conscious Change – Meditate before picking phone up in the morning, make it my first priority of the day.*

What Nurtures: How can I reduce my conflict right now? – *Naughty Notes – I know you are telling yourself there is no point, but you know this is nonsense and will pass like every other time - Conscious Change – Set a reminder on my phone that goes off every morning to allow me to journal/tap/explore how I am feeling before it escalates into something bigger.*

<u>What Nurtures: Are You Tapping on what niggles you before it gets bigger?</u> – *Naughty Notes* – *You are telling yourself you have tapped but it was ages ago and not on this topic either! - Conscious Change – Tap on whatever is niggling me every time I put the kettle on to boil. That will become my new tapping time.*

See how easy this is? What we are doing with the Thriving Guide is putting all your resources in one place as a reminder of what you can do for yourself each and every day, or at the very least when you start to feel low, but hopefully before you want to scream!

You already have all the tools you need to thrive, it's just you have spent a lifetime doing things another way, so this way may take some time to become a new and healthier habit for you.

Half the reason we relapse into any "bad" habits is because we forget what we already know helps.

CHAPTER 36
MY GREATEST TEACHER

My greatest teacher, without a shadow of a doubt, was my Chronic Fatigue Syndrome.

If it was not for getting CFS, I have no idea where I would be today, or even if I would be here at all.

I was slowly killing my spirit and body - it's no wonder I got ill. I burnt the candle at both ends, I was totally disconnected from my body, health, community and life. I wasn't listening to any whispers or even shouts from my body or life to make a change, and I thought I was invincible, even though I was ill a lot.

I just kept going, pushing, pleasing, achieving, not feeling enough, needing to do more and be more. I was pushing so hard to create what I thought would be a perfect life - a life where I'd finally be happy and feel alive - that I was slowly killing myself.

Then along came CFS and for the first couple of years, I was even worse than ever before because I believed the stories that you could not recover from it and that I'd be like this forever.

However, I started to notice its teachings, I started to realise I had made myself ill. Not that it was my fault - I believe it's actually society's fault. Society has us believe the more we work, the better homes and houses and material things we have, and the prettier we look, the happier we will be. It's always just out of our reach, making us push that little bit harder. But we get burnt out and tired of it all, so we self-medicate with drugs, alcohol, social media, TV, shopping, sex and anything else as a distraction. But this, although it numbs temporarily, usually makes things worse in the long run, adding to our pain and disconnection.

I started to see CFS as my teacher, my compass, my body showing me what had to change to be happy and healthy. And not one of these things was anything I had focused on before. It was not about being more, doing more or achieving more. It wasn't about who I was with or how much I earned. It was about that connection back to my body and life once more, no longer rushing on by, disregarding what was going on around me.

I remember the first time I decided I was not going to be jealous of the people walking past my window going to work, and instead, I sat at the window and watched the birds, butterflies and squirrels playing in the garden instead. And for the first time in a very long time, I felt totally blessed for CFS coming into my life. Wow, how much of life I had missed trying to create a life I thought I needed. All those people rushing to work were missing this - they we totally focused on getting to work, to make money, to fund the future "happy" life, rather than seeing and feeling life right now.

Over the following years, there were many ups and downs, but often each down became less intense and hung around for less time. It was because I started to be open to the learnings, the lessons in each thing CFS threw at me.

It is my belief that any long-term illness, trauma or bereavement can be our greatest teacher, if we allow them to be - or it can suck us under and be our greatest burden. It is of course totally normal to get sucked under some-times, we are human after all.. However, once we become aware of where we have been, then we can choose: will I allow myself to see the teaching or will I continue to feel sorry for myself and add to my burden?

It's up to you, you choose, but for me I had to keep choos-ing life. I knew that CFS was here for a reason, I knew society was not teaching us to be happy and healthy, far from it. So, CFS did this for me and now I pass on what it taught me to you.

CFS was my greatest teacher and probably saved my life (although for many years of it I felt like it had stolen it away). Even before CFS came along, I have never felt so happy, so healthy and so connected as I do since it has disappeared. It's given me the tools to really live, to really feel alive and to really embrace life, its lessons and its magic for many, many years to come.

Faith xx

PS: For an up-to-date list of my favourite inspiring books and films that helped me with my recovery, search for "inspiring" on my website.

CHAPTER 37
I DIED A THOUSAND DEATHS

I've died a thousand deaths, and will no doubt die some more

With each death comes release from
all that I am not and much more

I've died a thousand deaths, and will no doubt die some more

The pain in that dying hurts like f#@k, but it brings with it more
knowing than ever before

I've died a thousand deaths, and will no doubt die some more

For I wish to live a life freer than before

I've died a thousand deaths, and will no doubt die some more

For with death comes a life worth living, more than ever before

I've died a thousand deaths, and will no doubt die some more

I'd happily release every mask to live with
a little more peace than before

I've died a thousand deaths, and will no doubt die some more

To live a life where I am true to me is worth the
death of all that came before

I've died a thousand deaths, and will no doubt die some more

Because the death of all that is fake, all that is pushing and people-
pleasing, needy and over-achieving is a death worth dying for.

Lightning Source UK Ltd.
Milton Keynes UK
UKHW040637140920
369876UK00001B/69